The S
N

Dr Sallie Baxendale is a consultant   t
who has worked with people with memory difficulties in the
National Health Service for over twenty years. She is the
author of more than fifty academic publications on memory
function. Her work in this field ranges from the development of rehabilitation strategies to studies of the ways
memory problems are misrepresented in the media. She
currently works for the Institute of Neurology, University
College, London. The full version of this book, *Coping with
Memory Problems* (Sheldon Press, 2012), is recommended
on the Reading Well Books on Prescription for dementia
scheme.

Sheldon Short Guides

A full list of titles in the Overcoming Common Problems
series is also available from Sheldon Press, 36 Causton Street,
London SW1P 4ST and on our website at
www.sheldonpress.co.uk

Depression
Dr Tim Cantopher

Memory Problems
Dr Sallie Baxendale

Phobias and Panic
Professor Kevin Gournay

Worry and Anxiety
Dr Frank Tallis

THE SHELDON
SHORT GUIDE TO
MEMORY
PROBLEMS

Dr **Sallie Baxendale**

sheldon PRESS

First published in Great Britain in 2015

Sheldon Press
36 Causton Street
London SW1P 4ST
www.sheldonpress.co.uk

British Library Cataloguing-in-Publication Data
A catalogue record for this book is available from the
British Library

ISBN 978–1–84709–366–0
eBook ISBN 978–1–84709–367–7

Typeset by Fakenham Prepress Solutions, Fakenham,
Norfolk NR21 8NN
First printed in Great Britain by Ashford Colour Press
Subsequently digitally reprinted in Great Britain

eBook by Fakenham Prepress Solutions, Fakenham,
Norfolk NR21 8NN

Produced on paper from sustainable forests

Contents

Contents

Introduction

If you are struggling with memory problems yourself or are caring for someone who has memory difficulties, this book has been written to help you cope.

The book is divided into two parts. The first part explains how memory works and describes various aspects of memory function. The brain uses many different mechanisms to store and retrieve information and even in people with far-reaching memory difficulties, not all systems are affected to the same extent. The second part looks at some of the most common underlying causes of memory problems.

There are no silver bullets when it comes to improving memory function. This, as you will see, is a recurrent theme throughout the book. The strategies that can be used to cope with memory problems can be broadly divided into three groups.

1 *Those that deal with the underlying problem*. These strategies tackle underlying problems that are interfering with memory processing. There is a surprising amount that you can do, even if your underlying brain systems are damaged. (See Chapters 8, 9 and 10.)
2 *Internal strategies that you can use to exploit the way your brain works*. The second set of strategies focuses on ways you can get the most out of your memory to try to maximize the likelihood that new information goes in and is properly processed in the first place, and minimize the obstacles that might prevent you from recalling it fluently later.

3 *Outsourcing your memory functions to external agencies to reduce the load.* The final group of strategies involves taking the load off an overburdened memory system by using external aids (from the good old-fashioned calendar to the most complex interactive digital apps) to record your information and jog your memory for you.

This three-pronged approach is unlikely to solve all your memory problems, but it may go a long way to reducing the nuisance they cause in everyday life, and that reduction lies at the heart of coping with memory difficulties.

The hippocampi

Throughout the book, reference is made to the hippocampi (plural). The word is taken from the French word for 'seahorses'. The hippocampi are two seahorse-shaped structures in the brain that play a crucial role in creating new memories. There is one on the right-hand side of the brain and one on the left-hand side. It is still possible to form new memories if one hippocampus is damaged, but if both are damaged, severe memory problems occur. Generally speaking, large, plump hippocampi are an indication of a healthy memory system. However, there are many factors that have a detrimental impact on hippocampal health and that cause the structures to shrink. The second part of the book examines some of these factors and ways you can ensure your hippocampi stay as healthy as possible, including a healthy diet and regular moderate exercise.

Part 1
HOW MEMORY WORKS

1

Are you paying attention?
Then we will begin . . .

In 2008, a family home in Manchester was burgled early on a Saturday evening. Not that unusual perhaps, except that the burglar stole items from the room in which the whole family sat watching a talent show on the television. Every member of the family was so engrossed in the programme that they failed to notice someone coming into the room, taking their belongings and leaving with them.

It's tempting to think of our eyes, ears and brain as a kind of video camera, capturing everything we're exposed to in an objective, all-inclusive fashion. But in fact, everything we 'see' has already been filtered and edited by our brains, long before we consciously process the new information. All too often we see what we expect to see and just don't notice the other stuff going on around us. We have evolved this way for a purpose.

Without this in-built filter, it is extremely hard to concentrate on anything. Without our even being aware of it, our brains filter out the irrelevant stimuli in our environment and help us to focus on whatever we have prioritized for the moment.

This is the first stage in the memory process. To remember something, *we have to have paid proper attention to it in the first place.*

This may seem obvious, but a failure to attend to something in the first place underlies many of the most common memory problems that people experience. For example:

> *My colleague introduced his wife at the party and 30 seconds later I just couldn't remember her name at all. It was so awkward.*

Often we haven't given ourselves a chance in these situations. The information just hasn't been processed properly in the first place.

Memory tip: Remembering names

If you know you are about to be introduced to someone, consciously anticipate that you are about to be given that person's name. Be waiting for it. Then interrupt the introducer *as soon as you hear the new name* and use it. For example, shake the person's hand and say, 'Hello Jane'. This way, you have processed the name by saying it out loud while looking at the person.

> *I get back to the car park and just can't remember where I parked the car. Sometimes I just have to walk through the rows systematically until I spot it. It's so embarrassing.*

Once a complex activity like parking becomes automatic, it frees up our brains to do other things at the same time. Thus it is possible to park 'on automatic' and then lose your car in a car park. This tends to happen most frequently in car parks that people are familiar with. It's rare that people can't remember which car park they have left their car in, but the exact location of the car just wasn't processed properly.

Memory tip: Did I turn off the iron?

The same applies to the common problem of failing to remember whether you have done an everyday task, such as locking the front door or turning off an appliance. Often the reason we can't remember doing these things is that they are so automatic, we weren't really paying attention at the time. Again, there is a relatively simple solution. If, when you turn off the iron, you say *out loud*, 'It is Tuesday morning and I have turned off the iron', you should have little difficulty remembering the action a few hours later. It is important to say it out loud as this ensures that you pay sufficient attention for the action to be consciously registered. And you need to make it time specific (e.g. Tuesday morning, Saturday afternoon) as this will give the memory a context. This will help you to remember it later.

These common examples demonstrate that we have to *pay attention and process something consciously* if we are ever to have a good chance of remembering it later on. While it may sound obvious, it is this failure to pay proper attention to the things we need to remember that underlies many of the most common memory complaints we experience every day.

Encoding

The ability to take in new information is the first part of the memory process. Psychologists call this process **encoding**. Some people find that they tend to be better at remembering things that they have read or heard, than visual details. Psychologists call this 'verbal' information because it is generally conveyed in words.

Other people find that they are better at remembering things visually. Faces are a classic example. Apart from mentioning a few distinguishing physical features, such as hair colour, a beard or glasses, it is almost impossible to describe a person's face to someone else who hasn't met that person before.

Try it now. Think of an acquaintance of yours and try to describe his or her face out loud. It's very difficult, and it's unlikely that anyone listening would get a clear picture of the person you are imagining. Although technology has helped to improve things a little in recent years, our difficulties in translating complex visual images into words is the reason police 'photofits' of suspected criminals still tend to look more like characters from the *Beano* than real-life miscreants.

How to maximize your encoding

A number of active study techniques have been developed to help maximize the information you take in when you are studying.

- If you are listening to a talk or a lecture, there is no substitute for taking hand-written notes. Writing notes makes you pay attention and also ensures that information is processed more deeply than it is during passive listening. Lecture notes do not need to be legible to anyone but yourself.
- Using abbreviations can increase the amount of information you can take down. If u cn rd ths u cn lrn hw to wrt qckly!
- To commit the new information to memory, you should rewrite your notes as soon as possible after the lecture has finished. The information is processed more deeply if you write by hand.

- If your visual memory is a strength, use visual sketches and annotations and rearrange the information spatially on the page. This re-drafting should always take place in a quiet, calm environment. Even background music or having the radio on can be a distraction.

There are a number of acronyms that describe active study techniques to help commit written information to memory; these include the RRR (read, write, review) method, the PQRST (preview, question, read, self-recite, test) method (see <www.scf.edu/content/PDF/ARC/How_to_study_a_reading_assignment.pdf>) and the SQ3R (survey, question, read, recite, review) method. Or look at the Open University skills for OU study, reading and taking notes at <www.open.ac.uk>.

2

Memory myths

Once information has been processed deeply enough to be remembered at a later date, it's tempting to think that that's the end of the story. Unfortunately our brains don't work like that. Although it may not feel like it, your memories of the past are constantly changing and being modified by your later experiences.

I just don't understand it. I can remember my childhood as if it were yesterday, but ask me what I did last week and it's a real struggle to remember.

This is one of the most common complaints that psychologists hear in their memory clinics.

Many people are perplexed by the fact that their memory for events in the distant past appears to be crystal clear, like looking through an open window on to the scene. However, these childhood 'memories' have

The reminiscence bump

Over-rehearsal may not be the only reason why memories from late childhood are so accessible and appear so vivid. Researchers have coined the term **reminiscence bump** to describe memories from adolescence and early adulthood because individuals typically recall a disproportionate number of memories from this time compared to the rest of their lives. These vivid and varied memories are normally encoded between the ages of 10 and 30.

almost always been rehearsed and revisited hundreds of times over a lifetime, whereas what you ate for lunch last Tuesday probably hasn't occupied much of your time or attention since you ate it. We tend to remember the big events from our childhood: the birth of a sibling, traumatic accidents, seeing something out of the ordinary for the first time. Even with these special events we can usually only recall some key features later on.

Telling a story

As we rehearse and revisit these events in our minds and in conversation, their key features form well-worn anecdotes. After a few years, it is these well-rehearsed anecdotes that we remember, while very little of the original memory may remain. Since we rarely tell a story without a purpose, every time we tell and retell a story, we edit it slightly for the target audience, removing irrelevant material and adding further explanations where necessary. This editing and retelling adds a subtle layer of distortion, which affects the underlying memory of the event each time. Although there is sometimes an element of conscious exaggeration for dramatic effect, the typical distortions are largely unconscious, and become indistinguishable from the original memory for the storyteller, who absolutely believes his or her recall to be clear and true at each retelling.

Interestingly, once a false memory has been inserted into the original memory, it seems to stick there.

Schemas

There is far too much detail in everyday life for us to remember it all – we just don't have the capacity.

To cope with this complexity, we develop simplified, generalized representations of things based on our experience. These representations form from a very young age. Psychologists call these simplified representations **schemas**. Schemas effectively allow us to summarize events. They are really useful, because they don't take up much memory capacity, but they have a downside. We often mistakenly 'recall' events that never really happened, because we associate them with certain schema. This distortion has important implications for the validity of eyewitness testimonies in court cases.

In addition to shaping our memories of events, schemas also often fill in gaps in our recollections. When there are small gaps in what we see, we tend to fill in the gaps with pre-existing schemas for the event.

Psychological studies and real-life examples emphasize just how unreliable our memories are. Even when the brain is working properly and we have full confidence in our recollections, we will have seen what we wanted or expected to see and will have then organized the information in a way that made sense.

Memory tip: Improving recall

Fortunately there are some effective techniques that can be used to try to counter some of these natural biases and distortions to improve the accuracy of our recall.

Studies have shown that people's memory improves if they physically revisit the scene of an event. Features in the environment can trigger new recollections. And the sooner someone gives an account of an incident after it has happened, the more detail that person is likely to remember later.

3

You never forget how to ride a bike

Everything that has been discussed so far has been in the context of remembering things that have happened in the past. Psychologists call this kind of memory **episodic memory** – the memory for episodes. We can also think of it as autobiographical memory – the memory of things that have happened to us. While these kinds of memories make up the bulk of our personal recollections, there are a number of other memory systems in our brains that appear to work in quite a different way and that don't seem to be subject to the same distortions.

Procedural memories

The knowledge of 'how' to do something is stored in the brain in a very different way from our memories of past events. People often say 'You never forget how to ride a bike', and it's generally true. Once someone has mastered a skill, it tends to stay with them. Psychologists call this **procedural memory** – the memory needed to perform particular types of action or procedure. Procedural memories are processed in our subconscious; and whenever they are needed – from getting dressed to reading the paper, playing a musical instrument to driving a car – procedural memories are automatically retrieved.

Procedural memories are created through **procedural learning** – the repetition of an action, over and over again until it becomes automatic. The more complicated a skill, the more difficult it is to commit to procedural memory. Fortunately we do most of our procedural learning when we are children. The young brain is primed to make all the connections it needs to acquire new skills.

Sometimes a procedure or skill becomes so automatic that it's difficult to remember doing it at all. The

Psychological choking

Procedural memories are generally very robust and resistant, but they can be disrupted by very high levels of stress. This often happens when someone is required to perform the skill in front of other people. It is as if access to the procedural memory store is suddenly blocked and the person performs like a beginner again. This is often seen in the sporting arena where sportsmen and women appear to crumble as the pressure builds, and often end up just 'giving' the game to their opponents, to the incredulity of their fans. This phenomenon is often referred to as 'choking'. Psychologists think this happens because stress increases the performers' self-consciousness.

Choking is not limited to the sporting arena; concert pianists, public speakers and even us mere mortals can all experience a form of choking. A world championship doesn't need to be at stake. When stress levels are high, you may temporarily lose access to your procedural memory, blocking the ability to complete even simple tasks such as paying for shopping.

action becomes so automatic and unconscious, we do not process it sufficiently to enable us to recall it later. Most of us have experienced the momentary disconcertion where you go to do something, like locking the back door before you go out, only to find that you have already done it. The action was so automatic, you just didn't process it the first time. Similarly, experienced drivers may be familiar with the sudden realization that they have not been aware of a recent chunk of their journey.

4

Remembering to remember

In the topsy-turvy world of *Alice in Wonderland*, Alice is thrown into confusion when she meets the White Queen in the woods. Just after the Queen has explained the 'Jam' rule (for the uninitiated, it's 'jam tomorrow and jam yesterday – but never jam today'), she goes on to explain how memory works both ways. 'I'm sure mine only works one way,' Alice replies. 'I can't remember things before they happen.' The Queen retorts that 'It's a poor sort of memory that only works backwards.'

Lewis Carroll inadvertently touched on a truism in these words. We do rely on our memories reaching into the future when we need to remember to do something. Psychologists call this **prospective memory** – remembering to remember.

Prospective memory has three key features:

1 An intention to do something later; for example, 'I must post Sam's birthday card.'
2 A delay between forming the intention and actually carrying it out.
3 The absence of an explicit prompt indicating that it is time to carry out the action (like an alarm) – you just need to remember to remember, at the right time, in the right place.

Psychologists have estimated that at least half of our forgetting is due to the failure of prospective memory.

This isn't really surprising when you think about it. Our days are generally spent forming intentions and then acting on them. It's not surprising, then, that some of these intentions never get fulfilled. Prospective memories can relate to set daily routines such as taking medications at regular times, or to irregular one-offs such as posting a letter, attending a medical appointment or picking up a pint of milk on your way home.

Memory tips: Strategies for remembering to remember

- Up the ante – the more important something is, the less likely we are to forget it. If your daughter is getting married next Saturday, it is unlikely that you will forget to go to the wedding. One way of increasing the likelihood that you will remember to remember is to increase the importance of the event, and the consequences if you forget. Take the example of a hospital appointment. If you only envisage a failure to attend as a minor inconvenience to yourself, the consequences of forgetting the appointment will be less than if you consider the wider implications for the doctor who is waiting for you and the patients who could have been seen in your place.
- Visualizing an action, together with a clear statement of intent, can make it significantly more likely that you will remember to do something later on. So if you want to remember to stop off on the way home and buy some milk, you might visualize yourself driving towards the corner shop and pulling up outside. As you are visualizing this you can say out loud, 'When I drive past the pub I will remember to turn left to pick up some milk from the corner shop.' Studies have shown that

this joint approach of visualization and explicitly
stating intentions out loud is particularly effective
at helping older people to remember and act
upon their plans.

- Studies of airline pilot errors show just how
important interruptions can be in derailing our
intentions. Any kind of distraction or interruption
can lead to mistakes and errors. Just being aware
of this can help. Whenever you are interrupted,
recognize the fact. Mentally acknowledging 'I have
been interrupted', and asking yourself 'What was
I doing?' and 'Where had I got to?' can ensure
that you return to the correct place in a sequence
of actions and bring your initial intentions back to
the forefront of your mind.

- Probably the most effective strategy is to make
sure that you have plenty of prompts and
reminders. Traditional 'to do' lists are one of the
most effective ways of propping up prospective
memory. Apps for smartphones can also be very
effective indeed. All prospective memory tasks can
be reduced to just one action – remember to take
the phone with you. Some memory prompts, such
as drug wallets or tablet boxes, are physical.

5

When it all comes flooding back

Genuine memory difficulties can also arise when you try to retrieve information from your long-term store and your access seems to be blocked. The information has been properly processed and you often *know* it's there. You may be able to recall all kinds of peripheral details, but the key point you want to remember remains elusive.

Difficulties in recalling information you know you know can be incredibly frustrating.

What causes blocking?

Human memory works rather like a museum. If an exhibit isn't very interesting and it is never looked at, it may be moved to a back room or put into storage where it may fade and begin to decay. Eventually it may be cleared out to make way for more interesting exhibits. Psychologists think that this is what happens to old memories that are very rarely retrieved or revisited. This is beneficial as it makes way for more useful memories. Sometimes we can't retrieve information from our long-term memory store because only fragments remain, or it simply isn't there any more.

Often when we go to retrieve one memory, another similar one comes to mind and 'blocks' access to the thing we really want to recall. This becomes more common as people get older, partly because the memories of a lifetime have similar characteristics and begin to 'overlap'.

Memory tip: Retrieving blocked memories

Research has suggested that about half of all 'blocked' memories are correctly retrieved within about a minute of trying to remember. This process is quicker if someone is trying to recall something in a calm, quiet environment. It may not happen for hours (or even days) if you are trying to recall something in a busy, noisy environment and feel under a great deal of pressure.

Improving access: using sensory cues

Although we tend to relive our memories verbally, primarily by talking about them, a large amount of sensory information is also encoded and attached to our memories of past events, including:

- smells
- tastes
- sounds.

Exposure to these cues again, even after a long time, can often trigger **involuntary memories** – rich 'snapshots' of past events that suddenly burst into consciousness. Being in the same place, smelling the same aromas and tasting the same food will all help to bring back memories.

This phenomenon can be used to a student's advantage in exam situations. Revising in the same place that you will take the exam may not be possible, but it might be possible to pair a distinctive perfume or aftershave with the revision and the exam and to chew on the same gum, or suck the same sweets in both situations. Every little helps when it comes to easing memories from your long-term store.

Word-finding difficulties

Word-finding difficulties can be one of the most frustrating 'blocks' of all. Word-finding difficulties occur when you *know* what word you want but just can't quite retrieve it.

There are two useful kinds of memory jogs that may help to 'release' the elusive word:

- using clues that relate to the sound of the word, e.g. what letter the word begins with, how many syllables it has, what it rhymes with;
- using clues that relate to its meaning, e.g. clues related to the category or background of the word can also help to unblock it. For example, if you are trying to remember the name of an actor in a particular film, you can try to think about some of the other films he has appeared in and his co-stars.

If you are worried about word-finding difficulties in a formal presentation, it is often useful to write down the key names and phrases on a small cue card. Often just the process of writing these words down beforehand ensures that they remain accessible when you need to use them, and the cue card isn't actually needed. However, if you have it ready, it will also lessen your anxiety and reduce the likelihood that word-finding difficulties will occur.

In formal social situations, it may be that circumlocution is the only way around a specific word block.

Circumlocution is using many words for something, when a concise and commonly used word or expression already exists. While occasional word-finding difficulties are very common and nothing to worry about, loss of access to the words for common everyday items, or word-finding difficulties that significantly interfere with an individual's ability to conduct everyday conversations, may be a sign of something more worrying. (See Chapter 12.)

Part 2
HOW MEMORY GOES WRONG

6

Stress, anxiety and depression

It's almost impossible to over-emphasize the impact that stress, anxiety and depression can have on your memory function. Between them, these three states are responsible for the overwhelming majority of serious memory problems in otherwise healthy individuals. They also exacerbate memory problems in people with neurological conditions.

Stress and memory

Stress is distinct from both anxiety and depression. Stress refers to anything that puts a system under pressure and disturbs its natural equilibrium. In the case of the human body, causes of stress, or **stressors**, can take many forms, for example excessive noise, light or pollution, poor nutrition, obesity, illness or drugs that are introduced into the system. Probably the most familiar form of stress, though, is the psychological kind.

These forms of stress often merge into each other. Very high levels of stress can also be induced by life events over which we have little control; for example, illness and death in our loved ones, relationship breakdown and unemployment, not to mention living with a teenager.

The discomfort we feel when we are stressed is part of the human body's response to a perceived threat or danger. As soon as we become aware of a threat, or sometimes just the increased possibility of danger, our body reacts by releasing hormones such as cortisol and adrenaline, getting us ready for action. These chemicals make us more alert and physically prepare our muscles so that we are ready to either fight or run away fast. This is called the fight or flight response.

This leaves the body in an unbalanced, uncomfortable state. If the increased levels of adrenaline and other chemicals are not used to fuel a physical reaction, the high levels of these hormones racing around the body can start to cause physical damage. Most people are aware that perpetually high levels of stress play a significant part in the development of heart disease. Scientists have now found that high levels of cortisol, a key hormone released by the body during times of stress, can also affect the brain.

Acute stress

Although chronic stress has a negative impact on memory function, acute stress appears to have the opposite effect. Numerous studies have shown that when people are under intense pressure they are actually better at learning new information and committing it to their long-term store, particularly if it has an emotional component. This is why people are often able to give detailed accounts of highly stressful events, for example if they witness an accident or are involved in a disaster. Many often say it was as if the event occurred in slow motion, such was the vivid detail they could recall afterwards. This is sometimes called **flash-bulb memory** – as if the memory has been caught and captured on camera, such is its clarity.

Flashbulb memories: Where were you when . . . ?

Flashbulb memories are formed by a special biological memory mechanism, different from normal memory processes. The mechanism is only triggered by exceptional events. Immense surprise is also often a key characteristic. Personal flashbulb memories are usually centred on births, deaths and accidents. A number of events have been responsible for collective flashbulb memories, including the assassination of John F. Kennedy, the death of Diana, Princess of Wales and the terrorist attacks of September 11, 2001 in the USA. Flashbulb memories are very robust and resistant to forgetting. The most enduring detail of a flashbulb memory is where you were when something happened. While the vividness and detail of flashbulb memories in people with Alzheimer's disease does eventually fade, where they were when the flashbulb memory was formed is normally the last thing to go.

Unsurprisingly, there is also a downside to the brain diverting all its available resources to consolidating new memories when you are under stress. The retrieval part of the memory system becomes far less efficient. It's much harder to recall something that you already know when you are under pressure, than when you are not. This will be familiar to anyone who has ever had a bad attack of 'exam nerves'.

Even if it were possible, it is undesirable to eliminate stress entirely from our lives. At the right level, stress hormones can make us feel excited, even exhilarated. The key to stress management is getting the balance just right.

Managing stress

There is much you can do to reduce the physical stress on your body.

- Maintain a healthy lifestyle with a good balanced diet. Researchers in Sweden have recently found that people who are overweight in middle age increase their risk of developing Alzheimer's disease by 70 per cent compared to those with a healthy Body Mass Index (BMI).
- It is your reaction to an event that causes stress, *not* the event itself that is intrinsically stressful. Finding new ways to respond to events you naturally perceive as stressful can be difficult. Sometimes it involves undoing a lifetime of learning. There are many self-help books available on stress management and some are better than others. Meditation, relaxation techniques and learning to approach and think about situations in different ways can all be effective in managing stress.

Anxiety and memory

Anxiety and stress are closely related, and a state of chronic anxiety often results from repeated exposure to multiple stressors.

One simple rule of thumb that is used for distinguishing between stress and anxiety is to look at the order of thoughts in relation to feelings. In anxiety, unpleasant feelings often precede the thoughts that go with them. People with chronic anxiety often feel bad and then mentally search around for the thing that is making them feel anxious. Having found something to peg the feelings on, it can be hard to feel better, as the feeling remains even when the apparent trigger issue has been resolved.

Anxiety disorder is a medical condition that occurs when anxiety levels become so elevated that they begin to interfere with people's lives. Memory problems are a diagnostic feature of the condition.

How anxiety worsens memory

Worry is a huge drain on the brain's resources, leaving little reserve for other functions. Raised levels of anxiety have a devastating effect on working memory, the system that temporarily holds several pieces of information in your mind and allows you to manipulate them to solve problems or make connections. A deficient working memory impacts on almost every area of cognition. If you are unable to hold information and work with it at the same time, it will have a significant impact on your ability to take in and understand new information and plan and make decisions. As proficiency in these tasks decreases, so anxiety increases even further as you begin to worry even more, and so a vicious cycle is created, with greater anxiety leading to even greater memory difficulties.

To reduce the impact of anxiety on memory function, this vicious cycle must be broken. Anxiety disorders can be treated with cognitive behavioural therapy (CBT), an extremely effective method with proven results in this area. Your GP will be able to refer you to your local Improving Access to Psychological Therapies (IAPT) service with therapists who are skilled in breaking these vicious circles. Sometimes medication is used to reset the brain chemistry.

Mood and memory

Depression is the most prevalent mental health disorder in the UK. In addition to low mood, memory difficulties and problems concentrating are core diagnostic features of depression. They are part and parcel of the condition. Studies have shown that people with depression find it difficult to sustain sufficient attention to complete cognitive tasks. However, they find it much easier than healthy individuals to maintain their attention on negative thoughts about themselves. Researchers have shown that these negative thoughts hog the mental resources that depressed people need to function effectively. It is no surprise, therefore, that people with depression experience significant memory problems in everyday life.

Depression doesn't only reduce memory capacity, there is also evidence that the condition interferes with what people remember. People with depression appear to pay particular attention to negative information and are not able to properly process positive experiences. In laboratory tests where people are given lists of random words to memorize, depressed people tend to remember 10 per cent more negative words than positive ones. In real life, they tend to remember events that are congruent with their mood – that is, negative information and events.

How depression affects the brain

These changes in memory function are accompanied by changes in the brain. The hippocampi are particularly vulnerable to the neurotoxic effects of depression. The altered neurochemistry damages hippocampal neurons and causes the structures to shrink. The extent of the shrinkage is associated with the length of depression and the number of distinct episodes of depression experienced across a lifetime. The extent of the shrinkage is also correlated with the magnitude of associated memory problems. The smaller the hippocampi, the greater the memory problems, particularly in the learning of new information. Although some of the changes that cause the volume loss in the hippocampi are reversible, studies have shown that the hippocampi of people who have only ever experienced one episode of depression remain smaller than those in people of a similar age who have never experienced the condition.

As with anxiety, memory problems are an integral part of having depression. They are not a side effect or a separate entity. Effective treatments in the form of psychological therapies and medications for clinical depression are available. Generally, as an individual's mood begins to lift after treatment, so his or her memory problems subside, although some residual difficulties may always remain, particularly when it comes to taking in new information. Accepting that this is part of the condition is the first step to coping. Utilizing the strategies outlined in the earlier chapters of this book will help to reduce the nuisance of these difficulties.

7

Physical health and illness

Some illnesses and their treatments can have a direct
impact on brain function, and memory difficulties may
be a key diagnostic feature or a well-known side effect
of the treatment. In other conditions, memory problems may arise indirectly from the effects of pain, fever,
fatigue, and other general symptoms of just feeling
unwell, particularly in chronic conditions.

Certain conditions have a specific impact on
memory function. Some of the most common are
discussed below. The list is by no means exhaustive
and if your condition isn't covered it doesn't mean
that memory isn't affected. If you are worried about
memory problems, though, it's always helpful to start
with a review of your physical health and any medications you may be taking.

Diabetes

Diabetes and memory loss are closely linked. Memory
function can be acutely affected in hypoglycaemic
attacks (a hypo) when blood sugar levels drop too low
and the brain does not get enough glucose to function effectively. There is too little fuel to enable the
brain cells (neurons) to effectively communicate with
each other and so one by one, the cognitive systems
start to shut down. If blood sugars are not normalized,
the person may eventually slip into a coma. Poorly

controlled diabetes with perpetually high levels of blood sugar (hyperglycaemia) can also cause brain damage over time, which can lead to permanent difficulties in memory function. The hippocampus seems to be particularly vulnerable to damage in diabetes. Hippocampal shrinkage has been recorded in both elderly and young populations with type II diabetes.

People with diabetes are also at increased risk for both Alzheimer's disease and vascular dementia.

Vitamin B12 deficiency

Humans rely on Vitamin B12 to function properly. When levels within the body are only slightly lower than they should be, people can begin to experience exhaustion, depression and memory problems. If it is untreated, chronic Vitamin B12 deficiency can cause severe and irreversible damage to the brain and nervous system, and the associated memory problems can resemble dementia, as they become increasingly severe. The longer someone has the deficiency, the more likely it is that permanent damage will occur. It's not difficult to include sources of Vitamin B12 in a normal carnivorous diet, as it is found in many animal products, including meat, poultry, fish, seafood, eggs and dairy products. It is also usually added to fortified breakfast cereals. Most people who have a Vitamin B12 deficiency do so because they cannot absorb the vitamin from their diet for some reason, rather than because they are not eating enough of the correct foods.

There are many medical reasons for mal-absorption, including pernicious anaemia, surgical resection of part of the gut, infestation by parasites and rare hereditary conditions. Mal-absorption can also occur in chronic alcoholism. Fortunately Vitamin B12 deficiency can be treated and memory problems can often be reversed following treatment if no permanent brain damage has occurred. Even if neuronal damage has occurred, treatment, in the form of injections, sprays, patches or pills, normally stops the progression of memory decline.

Thyroid disorders

Symptoms of hypothyroidism can include fatigue, weight gain, poor concentration and memory problems. These problems can come on very gradually and people may live with them for many years before the problem is diagnosed. Fortunately hypothyroidism can be easily diagnosed with a simple blood test, and the treatment involves taking a simple supplement. Generally the memory problems associated with hypothyroidism fully resolve following appropriate treatment.

Post-operative cognitive dysfunction

Post-operative cognitive dysfunction (POCD) is the term used to describe changes in memory function that can occur after the use of an anaesthetic. People commonly experience mild memory difficulties in the immediate post-operative period as the anaesthetic wears off and strong painkillers are administered, both of which have a powerful influence on brain function. However, some people experience more long-term problems with memory function after surgery.

Chemotherapy

Many people undergoing chemotherapy for cancer experience a sort of mental fog during and after the process, and these memory difficulties are often referred to as 'chemo-fog' or 'chemo brain'. Common problems include an inability to sustain concentration, word-finding difficulties, slowed-up thinking and trouble multitasking. These symptoms can be extremely distressing and hard to cope with, particularly as they tend to come hard on the heels of all the other difficulties a diagnosis of cancer brings. Estimates of the percentage of people who suffer 'chemo brain' vary widely, ranging from 15 per cent to 70 per cent in medical studies.

It is important to remember that not all memory problems in those with cancer are caused by chemotherapy. One study found similar levels of memory problems in a group of people with cancer who didn't undergo chemotherapy. Memory problems can be caused or exacerbated by many features of having cancer, including the cancer itself, exhaustion, sleep problems, depression, stress and anxiety. Other drugs used as part of treatment, such as steroids, anti-nausea medications, drugs used for surgery or pain medicines, may also be responsible for memory problems in these people.

Neurological conditions

Every neurological condition has the potential to affect memory function since, by definition, neurological conditions are the result of brain dysfunction at some level or other. Sometimes this dysfunction may fluctuate and be temporary, for example in certain types of multiple sclerosis (MS) and epilepsy. In other conditions, such as a traumatic brain injury or a stroke, the underlying damage or dysfunction may be stable but permanent.

Psychiatric conditions

There is an increasing overlap in our understanding of psychiatric and neurological conditions, and how the two kinds of condition may interact. The last decade or so has seen increasing interest in neuropsychiatry, which explores the common ground between mental disorders and diseases of the nervous system. Sophisticated scans have revealed structural and chemical abnormalities in the brains of people who experience psychiatric illness, and the lines of distinction between the two medical specialties have become increasingly blurred as a result. It follows then that the disturbances in thought and behaviour that accompany psychiatric illness often have a significant impact on memory function. It is also the case that external strategies – memory aids such as routines, apps, diaries and to-do lists – tend to work better than internal ones in this group. However, when behaviour and thoughts are very disturbed, for example in acute psychiatric conditions, it is often difficult to implement methodical routines, and as with neurological conditions, an acceptance of memory problems as part of the condition is necessary.

8

Diet and exercise

Although your brain makes up only about 2 per cent of your body mass, it uses approximately 20 per cent of your oxygen consumption every day. It needs the right fuel to function effectively. This is influenced to some extent by diet, but the delivery system also has to be effective.

To view brain function as separate from other vital organs when it comes to fitness is therefore a mistake.

Walk yourself to a bigger brain?

A group of researchers from America scanned 120 older adults, aged between 60 and 70, and measured their hippocampi. Half of the subjects were then enrolled on an exercise programme whereby they walked for 40 minutes, three days a week. One year later, the people who had completed the walking programme had increased their hippocampal volumes by 2 per cent, effectively reversing age-related volume loss by one to two years. These volume increases were also accompanied by improvements on memory tests.

It's never too early to benefit from exercise from a memory perspective. Exercise in mid-life is also associated with a decreased risk of developing dementia in older age. Some studies have estimated that the risks are reduced by up to one-third. Walking just one mile a day (perhaps to the local shops and back) can make all the difference.

Your brain health and function are closely linked to your physical condition. It follows that exercise and physical fitness have a significant effect on memory function.

Obesity

Obesity has now reached epidemic proportions, with 60 per cent of the UK adult population classified as overweight. One in four adults is obese (i.e. has a BMI of over 30). Over 30,000 people die in the UK every year from causes that are directly attributable to obesity. This means that obesity-related deaths account for 6 per cent of all recorded deaths every year. Sadly one-third of these people die before the age of 65.

Obesity in middle age is not only associated with an increased risk of developing dementia in old age. Middle-aged people who are obese have more memory problems than those of a similar age and background who are a healthy weight. They also have smaller hippocampi. Where you carry your excess weight also has a significant influence on hippocampal health. One study found that central obesity (classic 'apple' shapes who carry their weight around their middles) is particularly damaging for the hippocampi. Studies have shown that the larger someone's waist to hip ratio is, the smaller their hippocampi tend to be. Apple-shaped individuals are at increased risk of developing cancer, cardiovascular disease and memory problems. Unfortunately we can't choose where we store excess weight, but if you are apple shaped and tend to gain weight around your middle, conserving your hippocampal health is yet another reason to keep your weight under control.

Obesity is also associated with a much faster age-related decline in memory efficiency. In 2012, doctors reported the results of a study that had tracked a series of over 6,000 people across a ten-year period. The study recruits were given three memory and cognitive tests over the course of the decade. The decline in performance on the tests was 22 per cent faster in the people who were obese compared to those with a normal healthy weight.

Lose weight, improve memory

The good news is that memory problems reduce (along with BMI) with weight loss. Scientists in Sweden tested a group of 20 overweight women on memory tests before assigning them to two different kinds of diet. One was 'the caveman diet' – a diet based upon foods that our early ancestors would have eaten: nuts and seeds and no processed foods. The second group followed a standard, low-fat, balanced diet. Both groups lost weight and both performed much better on the memory tests after six months of successful dieting.

Diet

Any diet that results in weight loss in the overweight has a good chance of improving memory function. But it is clear that some diets are associated with accelerated damage to brain cells, in particular the brain cells in the hippocampi. A high intake of saturated fats and simple carbohydrates is not only linked with the development of obesity and an increased risk of Alzheimer's disease. It is correlated with biological changes in the hippocampi well before the development of Alzheimer's disease.

Some scientists have even argued that the hippo-campal dysfunction caused by this kind of diet interferes with our ability to stop ourselves from responding to environmental cues associated with food, ultimately making us eat more than we need when food is plentiful and so creating a vicious circle. The more saturated fat and sugar we eat, the more likely we are to lose touch with feelings of hunger and satiety. We then begin to eat in response to external cues, primarily the availability of food and the amount on our plates.

Many people are already aware of what constitutes a healthy diet. It's sticking to it that is the problem. This is partly due to the long-term nature of dietary changes required for success and the lack of immediate results. However, when it comes to memory function, many people do report a 'clearing' of their minds within just a few days of beginning a low-fat, low-carbohydrate regime. You have nothing to lose (except weight) and everything to gain with this approach.

9

Hormonal changes

The correct balance of oestrogen, progesterone, testosterone and thyroid hormones are essential for maintaining cognitive functions. The concentrations of these hormones are often higher in the brain than they are in the bloodstream. Some brain cells actually produce their own supply of these hormones. It follows, then, that hormone imbalances can have a dramatic effect on brain function.

Memory and the menstrual cycle

Many women experience regular changes in mood at certain times in their menstrual cycle. There is a large amount of evidence to suggest that memory functions also fluctuate across the menstrual cycle. Women tend to perform better on tests of verbal fluency and on tasks that require fine motor skill in the middle phase of their cycle, while they perform better on tests of spatial ability during the menstrual phase. These fluctuations in cognitive performance are correlated with the fluctuating levels of estradiol (an important ovarian sex hormone) throughout the menstrual cycle. Though the results vary, and some people seem to be more susceptible than others, levels of estradiol are correlated positively with scores on tests of verbal fluency and negatively correlated with scores on tests of spatial ability.

Keeping a diary of memory lapses may help you to identify any cyclical aspects to memory problems, and you may be able to arrange important work/life commitments to avoid the times when you are more likely to struggle.

Pregnancy and childbirth

Many studies have found that pregnant women and new mothers perform more poorly in memory tests than women of a similar age who are not pregnant or who have not given birth. Some have argued that these memory problems are simply due to the stress and sleep deprivation associated with pregnancy and looking after a new baby. The physical stress of pregnancy on the body is huge.

There is also a growing body of evidence to suggest that the dramatic hormonal changes that occur in pregnancy and childbirth have a direct impact on brain function, particularly memory abilities. Again, some women seem more susceptible to these changes than

> ### Memory tip: Coping with memory problems following childbirth
>
> Memory problems after childbirth are difficult to cope with. There is so much new information to take in and new mothers are often in a perpetual state of exhaustion and anxiety. Accepting that these problems are common and finding support from other new mothers can be helpful. Setting up clear routines, accepting all the help you can get and not expecting too much of yourself, particularly in the early days, will also ease the burden on your memory, until things normalize again.

others. For most women, memory problems that come on during the final trimester of pregnancy tend to resolve over the first year of their child's life. However, there is some evidence suggesting that they may persist longer in women who undergo a very traumatic birth, where levels of the stress hormone cortisol are raised for a prolonged period, possibly causing some damage to hippocampal cells.

Menopause and post-menopause

In the UK the average age for the menopause is 52. A menopause that occurs before the age of 45 is classified as premature. As oestrogen levels decrease, menstrual periods become less frequent and many women suffer a variety of physical symptoms including hot flushes, night sweats, insomnia (sometimes exacerbated by vivid nightmares), itchy skin and mood swings. Women often notice an increase in memory problems during the menopause.

The risks and benefits of HRT

Studies have shown that hormone replacement therapy (HRT) can have a beneficial effect on memory function in some women, but the timing is critical. If HRT is initiated seamlessly with the onset of a natural meno-pause, and is taken for 2–3 years, it is associated with a decreased risk of memory problems in later life. Some studies suggest that these protective effects can last up to 10 to 15 years after the HRT has been stopped. However, when HRT is started in older women who have already been through the menopause it seems to be associated with a higher risk of dementia. There appears to be a 'healthy cell bias' in the action of oestrogen on the brain. When healthy neurons are exposed to oestrogen it has a beneficial effect on their survival, but it seems to exacerbate the demise of already compromised neurons.

After hysterectomy

The surgical removal of the uterus and ovaries effect-ively deprives women of several years of oestrogen exposure. Studies that have compared women who received hormone replacement therapy immediately after these procedures with women who didn't, found that HRT appears to protect memory skills. Long-term studies have found that women undergoing this kind of surgery who then took HRT until the age of 50 (the approximate time of the natural menopause) had no increased risk of cognitive impairment or dementia, and their memory skills were comparable to women who had undergone a natural menopause at 50.

10

Normal age-related cognitive decline

Although the human brain doesn't fully mature until our mid-twenties, sadly some functions have already started to deteriorate by 30! Age-related decline in cognitive function tends to follow a set pattern. These changes are thought to have some evolutionary advantages, with wisdom and knowledge superseding physical prowess as we get older.

Psychologists divide cognitive functions into different domains. The following are the four main abilities that comprise intellectual function – the way we understand and interact with the world.

Verbal comprehension

Verbal comprehension is a measure of how well you can understand and use language – for example, the extent of your vocabulary; how well you understand and can express abstract concepts; and general knowledge. As a rule, these abilities continue to develop throughout life, even into the seventh decade. Even in very old age (over 80) these abilities are generally preserved. Traditionally such abilities are classed as wisdom.

Perceptual reasoning

Perceptual reasoning is the ability to spot visual patterns and also to make sense of three-dimensional relationships. Reading a map upside down or being able to complete a Rubik's cube both require good perceptual reasoning skills, as does mastering an IKEA self-assembly instruction sheet. Although people with good verbal comprehension skills also tend to be good at these tasks, the two things don't always go together. Perceptual reasoning appears to peak early in life and proficiency remains relatively stable from the age of 16 to the mid-thirties. However, these abilities then begin a steady decline over the following decades into old age, with the steepest decline occurring between the mid-forties and the mid-sixties.

Working memory

Working memory is the ability to hold a piece of information in your head and manipulate it at the same time. Mental arithmetic relies on working memory, for example. We use working memory all the time to plan and make decisions, particularly when working on the logistics of any given situation. Working memory underpins many everyday tasks. Studies have shown that working memory skills are developed by the age of 18 and remain stable until the mid-fifties. They then begin to deteriorate gradually. Difficulties sustaining concentration and new difficulties in 'losing the thread' often begin to emerge in the mid-fifties. These difficulties are usually due to normal age-related declines in working memory.

Processing speed

Of the four principal intellectual domains, processing speed is the function that shows the most dramatic decline with age. Processing speed refers to the speed with which we can take in and react to information from the outside world. By the mid-fifties, slowing begins to manifest itself in everyday life. In busy environments, such as fast-paced work meetings, where there is a lot to take in, people may need information to be repeated, or they may miss key pieces of information if it is presented too quickly and they are still processing things that have been said earlier.

Memory tip: Coping with slowed processing speed

Finding ways to slow the rate at which information is given is the most effective way of dealing with this normal age-related decline. This may include introducing a clear structure to office meetings and ensuring that they are chaired competently, and recapping after every topic has been discussed. These strategies work well if they are in your control. However, for most of us they are not. Your next best bet is to outsource the recording of information as a back-up for your memory, which will allow you to digest the details at your leisure. Dictaphones, livescribe pens (<www.livescribe.com/uk>) and effective note-taking may be the answer.

Mild cognitive impairment

Mild cognitive impairment (MCI) is the name given to memory difficulties that are beyond those associated with normal age-related decline but that are not significant enough to interfere with an individual's daily activities. There are a number of different reasons for MCI, many of which are described in this book, but in elderly people MCI is often a precursor to dementia. When MCI is due to depression or anxiety and the underlying problem is treated, the symptoms can often resolve.

There are currently no proven treatments for MCI, although some studies have reported that people with MCI who regularly take folic acid and vitamin B12 supplements are less likely to go on to develop Alzheimer's disease than those who don't take the supplements. These vitamins are known to inhibit the production of an amino acid called homocysteine, and high levels of homocysteine in the bloodstream have been associated with an increased risk of dementia, so there may be something in it.

Memory tips: Slowing down memory decline

So can you do anything to slow down the inevitable decline in memory skills as you get older? The answer seems to be 'yes':

- Keeping your brain stimulated shouldn't be a chore. Read more books, play more games, complete puzzles. No one is suggesting you go back to school, but seek out something you enjoy, something that makes you think, and make sure that you find time for it on a regular basis.
- Learning a new skill seems to be a particularly effective strategy. One study found that learning to juggle increased brain volumes.
- For many people in full-time employment, their work more than meets their requirements in this area. It is therefore particularly important for people to think about how they will maintain adequate levels of mental stimulation as they approach retirement. The University of the Third Age (U3A) is a fantastic resource (see <www.u3a.org.uk>).
- There is also a lot of evidence that people who maintain an active social life tend to have fewer memory complaints than those who become isolated as they grow older.

11

Amnesia

Amnesia, from the Greek *a*, 'without', and *mnesia*, 'memory', refers to a total absence of memory. Short periods of amnesia occur when the brain is unable to process new information properly for some reason, usually through illness, injury, chemical imbalance or, very rarely, severe psychological trauma.

Neurological conditions

Many neurological conditions can lead to short periods of amnesia.

Epilepsy People with epilepsy are often amnesic for the events that occur during their seizures; if they have generalized tonic clonic seizures (the fall-to-the-ground, violent shaking kind) they are always amnesic for the event. There is however a rare kind of epilepsy called **transient epileptic amnesia** (TEA), where the only manifestation that something is wrong is that the individual is suddenly unable to remember things that have happened in the past – recent events from a couple of weeks ago or events from much further back.

Head injuries Generally speaking, the length of the amnesia correlates with the severity of the head injury; so much so that doctors routinely use the duration of **post-traumatic amnesia** (PTA) to assess the severity of the head injury the patient has sustained. PTA is the length of time it takes until someone who has had a head injury is able to start remembering things on a continual basis again. This is often long after the person recovers consciousness, and in very severe cases it can last months. People with such severe head injuries are sometimes unable to remember the events that led up to the accident. This is called **retrograde amnesia**. Like people with epilepsy, those who survive head injuries often experience significant memory problems once they recover.

More rarely, the brain's capacity to process new information can be permanently damaged. **Anterograde amnesia** is a condition where someone is completely unable to form any new memories at all.

Psychogenic amnesia

Psychogenic amnesia, though popular with Hollywood, refers to a very rare psychological condition where people suddenly forget all their autobiographical details. They normally come to the notice of the authorities when they are found confused and wandering, or on public transport, and are unable to give their name or address or any details about their previous lives. It is often difficult to discover their true identity, as these people tend to be found without any identifying information like a wallet or mobile phone on them. When they are finally reunited with their loved ones, they do not recognize them or anything about their previous lives. Medical investigations in these people, in particular brain scans, show no abnormalities. This kind of memory loss often afflicts fictional characters in films, but in reality only a handful of cases of psychogenic amnesia have been presented in the medical literature. Doctors still have much to learn about this rare condition, but the information we have to date suggests that it may be an extreme psychological response to a desire to change key aspects of one's life and to start again.

Korsakoff's syndrome This syndrome arises when brain damage occurs over an extended period of time in people with a long history of alcohol abuse; eventually it can lead to an inability to process new information and the development of amnesia. People with Korsakoff's syndrome have difficulties learning new information and recalling recent events. Sometimes large gaps in their memories for events from the past also open up, although their social skills and problem-solving abilities tend to be relatively unaffected. A common way of coping with these gaping holes in memory is to fill in the gaps with likely scenarios. This is called confabulation.

Dementia In dementia the mechanisms for encoding new information and those for retrieving old information are slowly eroded as the disease progresses (see Chapter 12).

Coping with amnesia

Establishing set routines can help to establish implicit memories in amnesic patients. With much repetition, people can sometimes be 'trained' to instinctively check a calendar every morning or in response to set cues such as meal times. Portable digital devices (such as tablet computers and smartphones) can also be used sometimes to set reminders and to store key pieces of information. These strategies are more effective in people with stable amnesia, rather than those with a progressive condition.

The charity Headway provides support groups for people suffering from amnesia following a brain injury and also provides support for carers. See <www.headway.org.uk>.

12

When to seek further help

Sometimes memory problems are a symptom of something more serious than just normal ageing. The World Health Organization (WHO) defines dementia as a syndrome in which there is deterioration in memory, thinking, behaviour and the ability to perform everyday activities. Although it occurs mainly in older people, it is not a normal part of ageing.

Alzheimer's disease

This accounts for approximately 70 per cent of all cases of dementia in the UK, and nearly 50 per cent of people over the age of 85 have the disease.

In Alzheimer's disease, the parts of the brain that process new information and commit it to memory are usually the first to malfunction. People often have significant difficulties remembering others' names and find it hard to recall recent events. Apathy and low mood can also be early symptoms.

The process may have started many years earlier. In the early stages of the disease, memory difficulties can be mild and many people are able to continue to live independently. However, as the disease progresses, people begin to forget things from their own personal history and lose the ability to perform challenging mental tasks – for example, counting backwards from 100 by 7 each time.

Eventually the gaps in memory and thinking become very noticeable. People may no longer be able to recall their current address or phone number and may give information from their past instead, for example their childhood address. They may also begin to lose very well-rehearsed information, such as the days of the week and where they are, particularly if they are presented with new surroundings, although at this stage they can usually still recall significant details about themselves and close family members, and can feed and toilet themselves.

In the final stages of the disease, people lose the ability to respond to their environment and are no longer able to speak, although they may still say individual words or phrases. They lose the ability to control movement and eventually swallowing becomes impaired.

Vascular dementia

The second most common form of dementia in the UK is vascular or multi-infarct dementia. This occurs when the arteries supplying the brain burst or become blocked, starving parts of the brain of oxygen, for example after a stroke. The factors that can increase the risk of vascular dementia are exactly the same as those associated with heart disease – high blood pressure, obesity, a sedentary lifestyle, smoking and a family history of vascular disease (cerebral or cardiac). While the risk of vascular dementia more than doubles in those with a history of alcohol abuse, consumption of one to six drinks weekly is associated with a *lower* risk of dementia among older adults compared to total abstention. As far as alcohol is concerned, it seems that a little of what you fancy may do you good, but moderation is the key.

Vascular dementia presents in many different ways. Memory functions can often be affected. It very much depends on which part of the brain each stroke damages. If the regions at the front of the brain are affected, someone may demonstrate impaired judgement or become rather disinhibited. Such people may make inappropriate or hurtful comments to their friends and family, and may not always realize that they have upset someone, or understand why someone would be hurt by what they have said. They may lose the ability to plan properly. Vascular dementia can often be distinguished from other forms of dementia by the 'stepwise' nature of the loss of function. People may find that they (or their loved ones with the disease) suddenly can't do something that they could manage the day before, or that a new symptom suddenly appears. In other forms of dementia these losses tend to be more gradual.

Other forms of dementia

Less common forms of dementia include conditions such as Lewy body disease, frontotemporal dementia or a combination of dementias.

People with Lewy body dementia often experience memory problems but also tend to have sleep disturbances, hallucinations and difficulties with motor coordination in the early stages of the disease, unlike those with Alzheimer's disease.

In frontotemporal dementia, areas at the front and side of the brain are particularly affected. Rather than memory problems, the initial symptoms may include personality changes and difficulties with language. There may be marked word-finding difficulties or difficulties in understanding what someone else is saying.

Although these different types of dementia have certain characteristic patterns in the early and later stages, there is a large degree of overlap. Recent brain imaging studies have suggested that these mixed dementias are more common than previously thought.

When to seek help

In an increasingly ageing population, dementia is a frightening prospect for both ourselves and our loved ones. The Alzheimer's Association have devised a simple checklist of 10 features that *may* indicate difficulties over and above those that would be expected given normal age-related changes in function.

1 *The extent to which the memory difficulties disrupt your life*. It is entirely normal to sometimes forget people's names or to put the kettle on and walk away. This tends to happen if we are busy and distracted. The information is not lost and we usually remember it later on. But if your memory problems are beginning to disrupt your life, to the extent that you need to ask for the same information over and over again, or that without family members to help you, you just can't remember what you need to do each day, then there may be a problem.

2 *Other cognitive processes being affected, as well as memory*. Some people find it very difficult to plan relatively simple tasks, like cooking a meal, or to solve logistical problems, particularly if there are a number of steps involved. Sometimes they just don't know where to start, or get lost in the

middle of a task. It's completely normal to make occasional mistakes when preoccupied and busy, but if you find it happening more often and that even simple tasks require a huge mental effort, and energy that you don't seem to have, there may be a problem.

3 *An increasing difficulty in being able to carry out familiar, routine tasks.* These can be domestic chores or leisure activities. Other worrying signs may be difficulties driving to familiar locations and periods of disorientation while out and about.

4 *Losing track of time.* Sometimes people find it difficult to remember the exact date or the day of the week. In later stages of the condition, people can lose track of the seasons or the time of day, and their sleeping/waking patterns can be disrupted as a result. However, there is nothing to worry about if you occasionally get the wrong day or are a couple of days out with the date.

5 *Difficulties making sense of visual images.* These include problems in working out spatial relationships between objects; problems in interpreting written text; and difficulties judging distances. These problems often come to the fore when driving at dusk, when people may find that they misjudge the speed of other vehicles or may miss unexpected obstacles altogether.

6 *Poor judgements in everyday life.* People can begin to make uncharacteristically bizarre, impulsive or ill-thought-out decisions, such as falling for scams they would normally see through. These decisions often involve financial transactions, and unfortunately criminals are all too aware of this. Online dating sites, for example, can ensnare the

vulnerable with scams conducted entirely online
under an assumed cyber-identity.

7 *New problems using words*. This is in addition to
normal, common word-finding difficulties. People
with dementia may call things by the wrong
name; for example, calling a 'pen' an 'ink write'
or a watch 'the arm time'. They may also develop
more general problems with conversation. These
can include trouble following the thread of a conversation, interrupting, or stopping mid-flow in a
conversation. There may be pronounced repetition
of stories and anecdotes.

8 *Losing things*. Not being able to retrace your steps
to find lost objects, or frequently finding things
in odd places (a phone in the fridge, cheese in a
drawer) may be a sign that something is wrong.
The frequent loss of objects can become very
confusing for people and sometimes leads to the
development of paranoia and the sense that other
people must be to blame.

9 *Withdrawal from social activities*. This is often due to
the difficulties described above, including difficulties in following conversations, loss of confidence
in driving and difficulties in making plans. It is
entirely normal to feel weary of work, family or
social obligations sometimes, but if this is a new
and pervasive feeling, something may be wrong.
Changes in this area don't necessarily signal the
onset of Alzheimer's disease. They are also seen in
depression. This is why depression will be one of
the diagnoses that a doctor will want to rule out
before diagnosing Alzheimer's disease. As with
the other signs, the key word here is 'change'.
If someone has always found social obligations

trying, then a failure to engage in older age is not a worrying sign. However, if someone noticeably withdraws from activities he or she has previously enjoyed, something may be wrong and a trip to the GP may help to identify what it is.

10 *Changes in mood and personality.* It is unsurprising that, with all these changes, the personalities of people with Alzheimer's disease can alter. Previously easy-going, gentle people may become blunt, suspicious, fearful or anxious. These reactions are often more pronounced when the person is in unfamiliar places or situations. This is different from becoming 'set in your ways' and liking things to be done in a particular way. It is completely normal to be irritated when people don't respect this or try to impose their own routines on you, particularly when this is in your own home.

Further help with dementia

For more information, contact The Alzheimer's Society helpline, 0300 222 1122, or see <www.alzheimers.org.uk> or the Alzheimers Association, <www.alz.org>.

If you are concerned about progressive deterioration, do not put off consulting your GP. Ask for an extended or double appointment and take a list of some of your memory problems, and of any questions you may have. If possible, take a friend or family member with you to help.